# L A S T I N G

# L O N G E R

## The Treatment Program For Premature Ejaculation

## Dr. Sy Silverberg M.D.

# About The Author

Dr. Sy Silverberg MD graduated from The University of Toronto Faculty of Medicine in 1967.

He continued his studies in sexual medicine with Masters and Johnson, Albert Ellis and other pioneers in Sex Therapy.

He has conducted a private practice for more than forty years in Toronto, Ontario and Victoria, British Columbia, Canada.

He was certified as a Sex Therapist by The American Association of Sex Educators, Counselors and Therapists in Washington D.C. (AASECT), and by The Board of Examiners in Sex Therapy and Counseling of Ontario (BESTCO).

He is a Clinical Member of The American Association for Marriage and Family Therapy (AAMFT).

He was a Director of The Education and Growth Opportunities Program at York University.

# Dedication

*To my beloved wife Catarina*

*The love of my life*

*always and forever*

# Acknowledgement

I would like to thank Stacy Elliott, a colleague and new friend, for her generous help in reviewing and editing the medical/scientific content of this book.

I want to thank Nick Cornwell, an old friend, for his dogged commitment to making this work so presentable and readable.

My heartfelt thanks to Fran Bleviss, my sister, for her life-long support and editorial acumen in all my writing ventures.

**Table of Contents**

# INTRODUCTION

I would like to begin by telling you how this book took shape as an idea and how it has come to take its present form.

This is a revision of a book I first published in 1978. The changes I have made are the result of the lessons I have learned in thirty years of full-time practice as a sex therapist.

Having spent thousands of hours, helping men to overcome the problem of premature ejaculation I came to realize that given the proper information most men can resolve the problem themselves. In the vast majority of cases, the solution to the problem lies not in lengthy and costly psychotherapy, but simply, in unlearning some incorrect beliefs and learning some accurate information and techniques.

Let's make it simple. Five facts tell the story.

Fact 1 - Premature ejaculation is not a disease. There is nothing "wrong" with you.

Fact 2 - No man is born with the ability to control ejaculation.

Fact 3 - Ejaculation is an automatic reflex response just like urination.

Fact 4 - Learning to develop control means learning to control that response.

Fact 5 - Any man who has been able control urination (has been toilet -trained) as a child can learn to control ejaculation.

Sound too simple? Take my word for it, and this comes from forty years of practice, it is that simple!

"Simple" does not necessarily mean easy. It takes practice and it takes time. If you are prepared to make the commitment, you can learn to delay ejaculation for as long as you want.

I decided to make this information available to as many men as possible. So, rather than writing a lengthy book full of historical data, statistics, anatomy, physiology, psychology and entertaining clinical examples, I have chosen to present, in the least complicated way, only that information, necessary to understand the process of ejaculation and the step-by-step instructions for learning control.

I need to add that throughout the following pages, I will be referring to partners as women. That is purely for convenience. Everything I say is equally true for male partners.

I would also like to acknowledge, to the therapists reading this book that I have taken some liberty in simplifying some of the physiologic mechanisms involved in the complex process of ejaculation. Although, I have excluded some of the details, the information I do present is accurate.

My aim is to present the process in a way that will be understandable to the greatest number of people.

# PREMATURE EJACULATION - Q&A

Q. What is P.E.? (Premature Ejaculation)

A. Premature is defined as "occurring before the correct time". Trying to define a correct or "normal" length of time to maintain erection is impossible. It will vary from couple to couple as well as with each encounter. At times a "quickie" will be perfectly acceptable while at other times it will be disappointing.

The goal of every sexual encounter should be, that both partners have a satisfactory experience, regardless of how long it takes. When that does not happen, ejaculation has been premature.

Q. How common is the problem?

A. Extremely common. P.E. is the most common male sexual dysfunction dealt with by sex therapists. Considering that the average time for North American men from entry to ejaculation is two minutes, it would be fair to say that most men ejaculate prematurely.

Q. Will the old suggestion for controlling, which involves thinking about non-sexual things to distract yourself work?

A. For some men, this technique may actually delay ejaculation for a very short time, but at what cost? You are there to enjoy the sexual experience, not to think about baseball statistics or car crashes. So, even if this does work, it may make the experience better for your partner but what about you? In addition, if you get good enough at this technique, it will probably not be long before you start to lose your erection. Then you have two problems to resolve: premature ejaculation and erectile dysfunction.

Q. What about the sprays and lotions they offer in magazines and online?

A. These preparations are generally topical anesthetics. Like the injection your dentist gives you, they temporarily "freeze" the nerves, so you can't feel the stimulation. Although this may delay ejaculation for a very short time, what is the point? Everything I said in response to the last question applies to this. In addition to you not experiencing pleasure, this stuff can rub off on your partner decreasing her sensation and pleasure. Lastly, some men or their partners can have allergic reactions that may result in weeks of pain, swelling and itchiness of the genitals.
Don' t waste your money.

Q. What about the breathing techniques that are recommended on some websites?

A. Any breathing or relaxation techniques can be useful to help you get centered and focused on your body before you have sex. Once you start, however, concentrating on your breathing will just be a distraction, and will therefore have the same negative effects mentioned above for the distraction techniques.

Q. Is it true that some prescription medications will delay ejaculation?

A. Yes. Some drugs (mainly antidepressants) will retard ejaculation in some men. They are potent medications that can have serious side effects. Any knowledgeable physician will only prescribe these drugs as a last resort.

Q. Why don't we learn to control naturally?

A. Controlling ejaculation is not natural. First, there is no evolutionary background for control. Human beings are the only animals who wish to control ejaculation. It is a part of the system that is built into all animals for only one reason, which is, procreation. Perpetuation of the species is its only function. No other animals, are interested in delaying ejaculation.

They want to get their sperm into their partner's vagina as quickly as possible, before some predator or competitor attacks them. We are the first animals to want to prolong the experience. To want to enjoy the experience, not just get it over with as quickly as possible.

Second, for most men, earliest sexual experiences were with masturbation, and were almost always done in secret and done quickly, to avoid discovery.

Third, most early sexual experiences with partners have been in circumstances where speed was an asset not a liability. Back seats of cars, parent's living rooms, and prostitutes do not encourage lengthy encounters.

Fourth, and most important, nobody teaches their kids to control ejaculation. If we lived in a society where it was as important to teach boys to control ejaculation as it is to teach them to control their bladders, P.E. would not exist.

With these four factors operating, is it any wonder that most men are not able to control.

Q. How long will it take to learn to control?

A. As with any learning experience, different men will learn at different rates. If you practice daily it could be just weeks, or rarely, less. If you practice once a week it could take months. The key to learning quickly is working at it consistently. When you learn any skill, such as playing the piano or playing tennis, you need to spend many hours practicing before you can relax and enjoy it. The same is true of learning ejaculatory control.

Q. Do I need a partner to help me?

A. No. A man can learn to control the reflex by himself. When he carries it into a relationship, there are some exercises that will ease the transition. Contrary to the original findings of Masters and Johnson, many sex therapists, have found that learning to control is something a man can do alone.

Q. Are there any physical causes of P.E.?

A. Rarely acute prostatitis, neurological injury or taking decongestants may cause P.E.

Q. Are there psychological causes of P.E.?

A. In most cases no. The exceptions are men with severe psychological problems for whom P.E. is one of many symptoms. In the majority of cases the condition is simply the result of maladaptive learning, and there are no deep dark psychological problems. Of course, anxiety around being able to "perform", does impact the condition.

Anxiety and/or depression may not be the cause of P.E., but they may develop as the result. Fortunately, these conditions almost always clear up once control has been learned.

Q. Does having P.E. indicate a serious problem in my relationship or mean that deep down I really do not love my partner?

A. Not in most cases. In the men I have treated, most have had otherwise good and healthy relationships. Problems in the relationship may arise as the result of P.E., but they too usually clear up once control is learned.

Q. Should I see a therapist about this problem?

A. If severe emotional or marital problems accompany P.E., consultation is essential. In the majority of cases, following the instructions in this book will solve the problem.

Q. How do I find a qualified therapist?

A. The American Association for Marriage and Family Therapy at: www.aamft.org
The American Association of Sexuality Educators, Counselors and Therapists at: www.aasect.org
.

# HOW EJACULATION WORKS

Ejaculation is the result of muscles in the penis contracting rhythmically, which forces the semen out. Contraction of these muscles are triggered by a reflex. To better understand the things you need to learn to control this reflex, you have to understand how it works.

A reflex is defined as "an involuntary response to a stimulus". Which means that when a stimulus is applied to the body, it responds automatically. You do not have to think about it to make it happen. There are three parts to any reflex. First some sort of stimulus is applied to the body, which causes a message to be sent along the nerves to the spine. Second, the message is relayed in the spine. Third, a message is sent back to muscles, which respond. The brain is not involved in this process. It operates at a spinal level.

The most commonly known reflex is probably the "knee jerk". If you have not experienced it yourself in your doctor's office, you have probably seen it on television or in a movie.

The doctor has you sit on the edge of his examining table so that your lower legs are dangling over the edge. He then hits below your kneecap with a small rubber hammer, causing your lower leg to jerk upward.

In this case, the stimulus is hitting the knee and the response is caused by muscles in the leg contracting. With ejaculation, the stimulus is, sexual stimulation. Sufficient stimulation will trigger the muscles in the penis to contract and ejaculation occurs.

Sounds simple, right? Unfortunately it is not!

As I mentioned, the brain is not involved in a reflex. However, the brain can take over control of any reflex and prevent it from working correctly.

Let us go back to the knee jerk to see how this happens. When the doctor hits your knee, if you are not thinking about what is supposed to occur, every time he hits your knee, your leg will jump. You do not have to make it work, it is automatic. If however, you start to watch to see if it is going to work properly, there is a good chance your leg will not jump. Why? Because the reflex is no longer operating at the spinal level. Your brain has taken over control. You are not trying to stop it from happening, you are simply observing to see if it is going to work the way it should..

Breathing is another good example. If you are not paying attention to your breathing, you do not have to think about when to inhale and when to exhale. It happens automatically. But, what happens when a doctor puts a stethoscope on your chest and tells you to breathe normally? You start thinking about breathing normally, and of course, you can't.

So, once the brain takes over control of a reflex, it will not work properly. In some cases, the reflex does not work as with the knee jerk. In other cases, as with P.E., the reflex can be triggered before you would like it to be.

With P.E., there is one further complicating factor. Anxiety can also act as a stimulus to trigger ejaculation. It is almost inevitable that once you identify P.E. as a problem, you will approach sex worrying about whether it will happen this time. That means you are in your head, watching and worrying. That means you have two strikes against you.

Your brain is controlling the reflex and your anxiety is adding to the stimulation. When these factors are operating, you are virtually guaranteed to fail.

The pages to follow will guide you through a series of exercises designed to eliminate these factors.

# HOW DO I LEARN?

What exactly do you need to learn to have control? I believe there are two things.

First, and I do not know if anybody really understands how, by repeating the exercises over and over, you develop voluntary control over a function that was involuntary (a reflex) to start with.

Second, with practice, you learn to control the muscles involved, This is a process similar to swinging a golf club or a tennis racquet over and over. At first, you try to consciously think about all the things you should be doing, and then one day, after hours and hours of practice, you no longer have to think about making it work right - it just does.

If you are thinking that this will be a difficult process, you are wrong. It takes time and effort but you can do it. In fact, you have done it before.

When you were born, your functions of elimination were reflex. When your bladder got full of urine, a reflex was triggered and the muscles in the wall of your bladder contracted and emptying it. When you were ready you learned to recognize the signals from your body that told you that the reflex was about to be triggered, and you learned to control it. Part of the process involved learning to develop control over the muscles.

So you have done it before, and you can do it again. Learning to control involves becoming familiar with the messages from your body that tell you that you are getting ready to ejaculate.

As you learned to control your bladder, you undoubtedly had "accidents". That is, you did not realize you were getting to the point of no return, (the point at which you can't stop, no matter how hard you try).

The key to learning is recognizing the signals from your body that indicate you are approaching the point of no return.

In order to recognize the signals that tell you ejaculation is about to occur, it is helpful to understand that ejaculation consists of two separate parts. These parts occur so closely together that at it takes time to recognize them as separate. Look now at Figure 1, which will clarify this.

# Figure 1

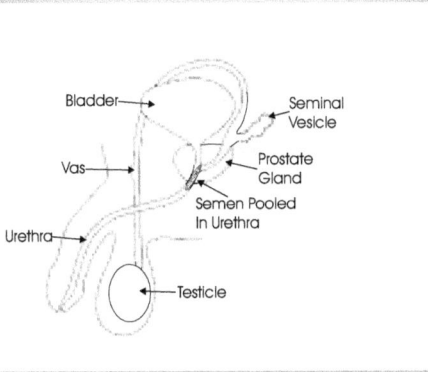

The viscous fluid that is expelled during ejaculation is made up of two components. The largest portion is called seminal fluid or semen. Contained within the semen are the sperm which are responsible for fertilization. Semen is produced in the prostate gland and the seminal vesicles. Sperm are produced in the testicles, and travel up the vas and mix with the semen.

The first part of ejaculation begins when the muscles around the vas contract, carrying sperm from the testicles to the urethra. At the same time muscles around the prostate gland and the seminal vesicles contract, forcing semen to join the sperm.

The first part of ejaculation is complete when this pool of sperm mixed with semen collects at the upper end of the urethra, just below the bladder.

The second part occurs when the penile muscles contract rhythmically, forcing this pool of ejaculate (semen plus sperm) down the urethra and out the end of the penis.

It is important to understand that while the first part is occurring, you can still delay ejaculation.

Once the second part begins there is no way to stop it, short of grasping the penis tightly, to prevent the ejaculate from leaving the penis.

This is something you should NEVER DO! This will only delay it for a few seconds, until you release your grasp. And doing this can cause serious damage to the urethra.

Learning to recognize the messages from your body that indicate the first part is occurring is the key to developing control. The sensations that occur during this first part are often described as a "tickling" feeling. It may be very subtle and hard to recognize, and some men are never actually able to clearly identify this sensation.

If you are one of those men who can't say to themselves, "aha, there it is", don't worry. Even though you may not be able to identify the signals consciously, with practice, you will pick them up unconsciously, and you will be able to control just as well as men who are aware of the sensations.

With continuing practice, you will begin to recognize (consciously or not) the signals from your body that indicate you are approaching this first part. When that happens, your control will be established. You will be able to come when you want to. In one minute or one hour, whatever the situation calls for, and you won't even have to think about it.

You will be in control, not the reflex and not the anxiety.

# THE ROLE OF ANXIETY
# IN PREMATURE EJACULATION

In order to effectively employ the exercises for learning control, it is essential to understand the ways in which anxiety contributes to the problem.

I mentioned earlier that the ejaculatory reflex can be triggered by anxiety alone. There have been many reports of ejaculation in situations of high anxiety without sexual stimulation. Teen-age students, for example, have reported ejaculation while writing stressful exams. The more anxious you are when you approach sex, the more likely you will come quickly.

There are two reasons for this. The first, is anxiety. The second is because you are in your head and not paying attention to the signals from your body that tell you that you are approaching the point of no return.

Let's look at where this anxiety comes from, as the first step to stopping it.

Boys and young men have always been exposed to totally unrealistic expectations of how they should be able to perform sexually.

In the past It has come from books, magazines and movies. Today with the Internet and the ready availability of pornography, the messages about how you "should" be able to perform are much more direct and graphic.

The message is: "If you are a real man, you should be able to get it up anywhere, anytime, with anyone, and keep it up for as long as you want. It should not matter how you are feeling, or how you feel about your partner. You should be able to perform this way every time you have sex."

This definition of "normal" male sexual behavior is absolutely ridiculous and completely unattainable. The only way to achieve that kind of performance is to divorce yourself psychologically and completely from the process.

Believe me, what you see on the Internet is a performance. These men become senseless and feeling-less in order to behave this way. They get nothing out of the act but a paycheck. They become robots or machines that program themselves to behave this way regardless of the circumstances, hardly something to aspire to in a genuine encounter with a partner.

Your behavior in any experience will depend upon many factors some of which include: your age, your health, your stress level in other areas of life, your level of fatigue, the amount of alcohol or drugs you may have ingested, certain medications you may be taking, your moral and religious beliefs, your feelings about your partner and your past experiences with sex.

I would like to expand on the very last point as it is of particular importance to our discussion.

If you accept that sex can be affected by many factors, you have to realize that throughout your life, there will be occasions when you will not be able to perform the way you would like to. If you hold on to the crazy definition of "normal" that I just outlined, there will be many occasions! I can guarantee you that every man will have experiences where he is unhappy about the way he performed.

If you accept that you are going to come away from a number of sexual experiences telling yourself that you have failed, how do you think you are going to approach sex next time?

You will be in your head, watching to see if it is going to work this time. Worrying that it won't. Not paying attention to the signals from your body. These are the very things that make certain that it won't. So, your chances of failing are even greater.

Every time you fail you worry even more, which just increases the likelihood that you fail once again. This becomes a cycle that perpetuates itself. Repeating over and over, getting more entrenched every time.

In some cases, the situation that caused the first failure, such as; drinking too much, being stressed at work, having the flu, or being overtired, may no longer be present. But once the "fear of failure" cycle has been started, it will continue until you find a way to stop it.

We will discuss ways to interrupt this cycle once we get into the exercises, but let us take a minute to look at how to prevent this cycle from getting started in the first place.

There is only one way to ensure that you never set this destructive, self-perpetuating cycle into motion.

Make sure that you never come away from sex feeling that you have failed!!

No, I am not kidding. This is something you can do.

# HOW TO HAVE FANTASTIC SEX
## EVERY TIME YOU TRY!!

How many times have you read a heading like this in magazines or books? "Give your woman toe curling, screaming orgasms every time. Just follow these simple steps". How many times have they delivered what they promised? The usual advice doled out in these articles is a series of "tricks" or techniques that promise you the perfect experience every time.

Let me save you a lot of money and frustration. The promise of perfect sex always, is impossible to achieve. Pursuing it will only lead to disappointment.
I am sure you know that you will not always have a great game on the golf course or the tennis court. You may be disappointed with those days, but you will not get down on yourself and start questioning your masculinity and your worth as a human being. You have not been taught to believe that having a bad day at one of these games makes you a failure.
Unfortunately, you have been taught this about sex. In order to develop a sex life where both you and your partner can come away from every experience feeling good about it and feeling good about each other, you must re-

educate yourself so that your expectations are realistic.

As I said earlier, the danger with holding on to this "normal" image of what it is to be a real man, is that, you are doomed to failure some of the time. The truth is, that even if you can live up to this ideal most of the time, there will still be times when your partner does not have a great experience, for reasons that have nothing to do with you (fatigue, stress, ill-health etc).

So, you not only have to give up your longing to be a super-stud, but you have to understand that you are not totally responsible for your partner's satisfaction. Providing her with the kind of stimulation she lets you know she wants, is all you can do. The rest is up to her.

I have spent a lot of time telling you about unrealistic goals that will doom you to failure and lead to your getting caught up in the destructive fear of failure cycle. Lets now look at developing some healthy, achievable goals.

If you continue to hold on to any goal, other than the one I am about to suggest, you are bound to fail some of the time. If you accept it you can't possibly fail.

Pay attention now! This is probably the single most valuable piece of advice you are ever going to get to ensure that you thoroughly enjoy sex for the rest of your life. Please do not just gloss over this.

Read the next line at least three times, memorize it, repeat it to yourself every day for the next week and really think about what it means.

THE ONLY REALISTIC GOAL OF ANY SEXUAL ENCOUNTER IS THAT IT BE A SATISFACTORY ENJOYABLE EXPERIENCE FOR BOTH PARTNERS, **NO MATTER WHERE IT ENDS UP**.

The last six words are the most important. They mean that regardless of whether the experience ends up with intercourse and orgasm for one or both partners, or an orgasm with intercourse for one partner, and for the other with manual or oral, or self-stimulation, or with the help of a vibrator. Or it may mean an orgasm for one partner but not the other. As long as you agree about a satisfactory end point, you can't fail.

The only way to make sure that one of these options is satisfactory and acceptable, to your partner is to be able to discuss it with them. To let them know, in the moment, what is going on for you and to find out what is going on for them. Then you can decide on how to finish so that you are both OK with it.

You do not have to pretend that it was an ideal experience if it was not. You can acknowledge that it was as good as it could be under the circumstances. In that way you can feel good about it and look forward to the next one, which will hopefully, (but not necessarily) be better.

We all have our preferences and I am not suggesting that you alter them or give up on working towards them. You know how you would like things to work out ideally. When you understand that it will not always end up that way, for a multitude of reasons, and when both partners are willing to accept that fact, then you can decide how to finish any experience in a way that is satisfactory for both of you.

This brings up another myth that can get in the way. For sex to be good, it should be totally spontaneous. You should not have to talk about it - that spoils it.

Can you imagine working out other problems that arise in relationships without words? Deciding what movie to go to, where to eat, what color to paint the wall etc. No one has trouble accepting that in a relationship, you have to discuss and negotiate decisions so that both partner's feelings and needs are taken into account. Yet, with sex, as a man you are supposed to know exactly what your partner likes and wants, and if she has to tell you, that is putting you down, emasculating you. Sounds pretty stupid when you spell it out, doesn't it?

Men of my generation (I am 68) seem to have more difficulty with intimate communication than younger men. I imagine that the most of you reading this book will fall into the latter category, so it should be easier for you. But, it may still be uncomfortable and embarrassing to talk openly about your insecurities in the sexual area. Yet you must, if you hope to get the most out of sex.

I am often asked, "When is the best time to bring this up with a new partner"? My answer is always the same. Before you have sex for the first  time. This sounds like a pretty radical thing to do, and you are probably worried that doing it will scare off a lot of potential partners. In fact, most partners will really appreciate your honesty and will respond very positively.

Am I suggesting that every time you meet a woman you immediately blurt out, "I have a sexual problem", of course not. However, when you get to the stage where things are going to progress beyond kissing, you can save yourself a lot of trouble, and dramatically increase the odds of things working out, if you follow this advice.

I would start with something like; "This is a bit embarrassing, and I know it doesn't sound 'cool', but, I have to let you know that I am the kind of guy who has to be very comfortable with a partner before I can function well sexually." That will open the door to discuss your concerns about coming too quickly.

Before you can do this with a partner, you must first acknowledge to yourself that you do need to feel comfortable with a partner before you can be at your best. And that this does not make you a failure.

This says absolutely nothing about your value as a man. In my practice, I have met many men who, in spite of outwardly presenting the ideal "macho" image, struggle with this. Professional football players and hockey players are prime examples.

Accepting this about yourself does not make you less of a man. If anything, having the guts to acknowledge that you do not live up to the ridiculous image that has been presented to you as "normal', takes a lot more courage than pretending you do. It also makes it possible for you to make the changes you want.

You are probably saying to yourself that all this may be true but there are still a lot of women who, if you approach them the way I am suggesting, will just laugh at you and say something like, "get lost loser".

The truth is that most women will respond positively. If you have a good female friend that you are not sexually involved with, read her these paragraphs and see if she doesn't agree. I would guess that there may one or two percent of women who "just want to get fucked", and will not be receptive to talking about sex. If you meet one of them, do yourself a favor, and say goodbye. With the kind of pressure they bring to a relationship, you are going to have trouble.

And realize that this is their problem, not yours. Things will not work out with them so save your self the pain and upset. There are far more women out there who will react with understanding and cooperation.

I know that, you are anxious to get on to the exercises but before we do there is one final bit of physiology that we need to look at.

Understanding this material will make the learning process a lot easier.

# THE SEXUAL RESPONSE CYCLE

You need to understand what goes on in your body as you go through a sexual cycle. I will describe the differences between the way a man who has control and a man who does not go through a sexual experience.

In the late 1950s and early 1960s, Masters and Johnson studied the physiological changes that men's and women's bodies go through as they are stimulated sexually. They found that the stages are basically the same for both sexes although, of course, there are differences because of anatomy. The researchers also found that the responses are the same regardless of the type of stimulation the men and women received. Their examination of approximately ten thousand experiences led them to distinguish four stages.

They called these stages "The Sexual Response Cycle" Figure 2 is a graphic representation of these stages.

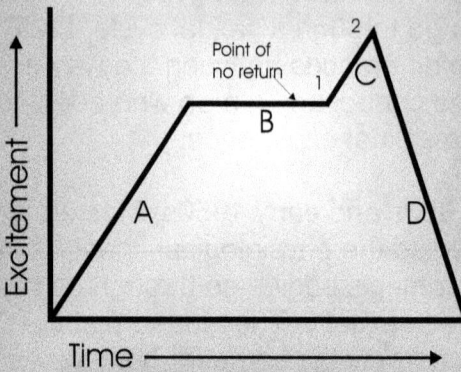

Figure 2

The first stage, labeled "A" in the figure, is called the "excitement stage" and begins when stimulation starts. As you can see, as the length of time that stimulation is applied increases, the level of excitement climbs. In both men and women, a reflex is triggered by the stimulation.

As you now know with all reflexes a message is sent to the spine where it is relayed and a message sent back to muscles. In this case the muscles are the ones that surround the blood vessels in the pelvis. These muscles relax which causes the blood vessels to dilate - get wider. That means more blood can flow into these vessels in the pelvis.

Page 36

This process is identical to the one that occurs after you have a meal and more blood goes to your stomach to help with digestion. Or when you are exercising, more blood goes to the muscles you are using. In preparation for sex, more blood goes to the pelvis.

The extra blood that flows into the pelvis of a man then flows into the penis. Because the inside of the penis is made up of sponge-like tissue, it absorbs the blood and becomes swollen and the penis gets hard and erect.

In a woman the extra blood flows into vessels that surround the vagina, and fluid passes from these vessels through the wall of the vagina to produce vaginal lubrication.

Now look at the third stage, "Orgasm", labeled C. This stage is also mediated by a reflex. It works this way. As stimulation continues a message is sent to the spine where it is relayed and a message is sent back to muscles in the pelvis, which contract rhythmically.

In men, muscles in the penis contract causing the pooled semen in the urethra to be ejaculated from the end of the penis (the second part of ejaculation). In women muscles that surround the vagina contract rhythmically.

You may have noticed that I jumped from stage one to stage three. Now, let's look at stage two of the cycle. It is labeled B and is called the " Plateau" stage. It is this stage that is most important to understand in order to learn to develop control. Figure 2 illustrates a man who can control. Notice that both his excitement stage and his plateau stage are quite long.

Now compare that to figure 3, which illustrates a man who is not able to control. He has a very short excitement stage and almost non-existent plateau stage.

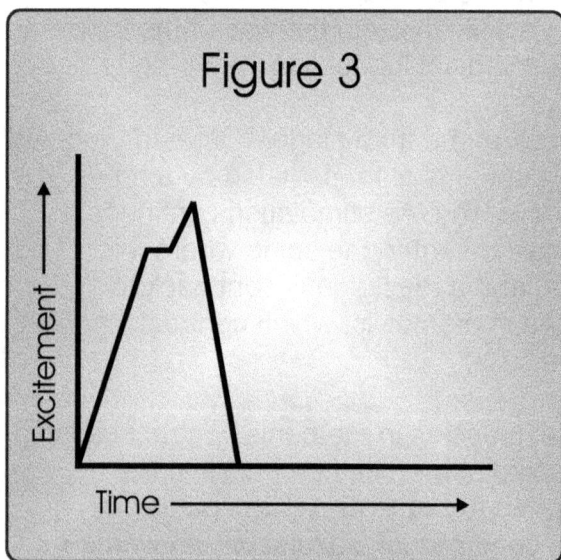

Figure 3

Recall our discussion of the two parts of ejaculation. First, pooling of semen in the upper urethra and second its expulsion from the penis. It is during the plateau stage that the pooling takes place. At this point you have reached the point of no return. Ejaculation will follow immediately. There is nothing you can do to stop it.

In order to be able to control ejaculation, you must be able to recognize when you are approaching this point. The exercises to follow are designed to help you do this.

The exercises are divided into two sections. The first is called "Solo Exercises" and the second, "Partner Exercises". If you have a partner who is anxious to start working with you immediately, it will be tempting to skip the solo exercises and start with your partner.

I want to stress in the strongest possible terms that this would be a mistake. If you do so, you will probably see some improvement but it is likely that your progress will occur more slowly and your ultimate degree of control will be less.

If you truly want to develop control, and by that I mean: you come when you want without having to think about it, I encourage you to follow the steps as outlined.

You can walk onto a tennis court and keep hitting the ball, until you are able to keep it in play. On the other hand with lessons that teach you the proper strokes and regular practice, you will end up a far better player.

Solo lessons means exactly what you think it does. Working on it alone. Masturbating!

Depending on your age, your up-bringing, your religious beliefs, and your partner's attitude, this suggestion may be perfectly acceptable or totally unacceptable. If you are in the latter group, you have been exposed to and taught many negative and untrue messages about masturbation.

Let me assure you, right now, that it will not ruin your vision, give you warts, make you "mental", or drain away your precious sexual energy. There is no longer any doubt among doctors and therapists that the supposed negative effects of masturbation are false. It is a perfectly normal and healthy form of sexual expression. Ninety-five percent of men begin to masturbate at puberty, and many continue to do so throughout life without negative consequences.

Attitudes have changed as more couples include masturbation in their lives. Masturbation only becomes a problem if it becomes a substitute for other forms of sexual activity.

Religious convictions are another matter, since some faiths still consider masturbation a sin. I do not feel it is my place to dispute or counter people's beliefs. I can only point out the fallacy of the old myths and indicate the advantages it can offer as a learning tool. Whether you feel comfortable in including the solo exercises in your program is a decision that only you can make. Let me point out what I see as the advantages to including it.

1. I must emphasize once again the importance of working at the program regularly. My recommendation is daily. It is totally unrealistic to expect a partner to be available or interested in working with you that often. So, even if you have a cooperative partner, there will be times you must work alone.

2. It is far easier to train your mind to focus completely on your physical sensation and not to wander when you are alone.

3. When you are working with a partner, it is very difficult to not be concerned with how they are feeling about the process. Are they bored, turned off, resentful? Usually none of these are true, but it is extremely hard to focus your attention on your body when a part of your mind is concerned about your partner.

## SOLO EXERCISES

If you have decided to work by yourself, we can finally begin the exercises.

There are a few important points to consider before you start. If you have been masturbating for some time, you will have developed a pattern that works best for you. Some of those patterns may slow down the learning process.

Many men rely on visual stimulation, such as the Internet to provide excitement. Continuing to do so during this process will definitely slow the learning down and may even prevent you from gaining good control. When you are viewing pornographic material, you are in your head. In order to learn most quickly, you must shift the focus to your body, to the pleasurable sensations produced by your sense of touch.

You are going to get tired of hearing me say it, but, the most important thing you can do to facilitate learning, is to concentrate on the pleasurable physical sensations from the nerve endings in your skin. You have to get "out of your head and into your body".

Another factor that may be a problem for you is the excessive use of fantasy, although some may be necessary to start with.

You can gradually decrease the amount of fantasy you use. It may take a while to make the shift because you will naturally drift into fantasy without even realizing it. You will have to work at catching yourself. Every time you realize you have drifted into a fantasy, you just say to yourself. "Whoops, there I go again", and gently bring your attention back to your body.

The key to developing control is recognizing the signals that show you are approaching the point of no return. You can't do that if you are in your head enjoying a fantasy.

You will probably have to use some fantasy to maintain interest and excitement, but you must shift the balance away from fantasy to touch.

I pointed out earlier that the ejaculatory reflex can be triggered by anxiety. I recommend that when you practice, that you eliminate all potential sources of anxiety.

Choose a time and place where you do not have to keep one eye on the door for anyone who might interrupt. And, do not practice immediately after you have come out of a stressful situation, with your partner, your boss, your bank manager or anyone else.

One final thing. This is where breathing exercises can come in handy. Before you begin, spend a few minutes in a relaxed position, just paying attention to your breathing.

Try to imagine that each time you inhale, you can see the air traveling into your lungs as a white light. Imagine you can see the air leaving as a blue light that carries out with it all the anxiety and tension in your body. Spending three to five minutes with this before starting the exercises will help you concentrate.

Please practice each step until you have achieved the goal it sets out. Follow the steps.

Only you can judge how long each will take. You will be tempted to skip some steps. Trust me that will not help you in the long run.


## SOLO EXERCISES

### Step 1

Begin to stimulate yourself in your usual manner. Do not make any special effort to delay ejaculation, but do begin to pay attention to the physical sensations in your penis and pelvic area.

Focus on the nerve endings in your skin and try to use fantasy as little as possible.
As you approach ejaculation, pay particular attention to what is happening in your body.

Imagine your self moving along the curve in figure 2, going through the excitement stage, plateau, with its two parts, and ejaculation. The goal of this exercise is to help you to begin to recognize the "tickling" sensation that occurs before ejaculation.

Be aware that although most men describe the sensation as tickling, you may experience it differently. With practice, you will come to recognize it. The next step is to begin to recognize the feelings that occur just before the "tickling". A point at which you can still stop ejaculation. Continue with this exercise until you are able to recognize the tickling".

Do not worry if you can't recognize these sensations. You will with repetition. In fact, some men are never able to clearly identify this first part at a conscious level, but with time, they recognize it unconsciously.

## Step 2

Begin stimulation until you have an erection, so that you are in the early excitement stage and nowhere near the point of ejaculating. Now discontinue the stimulation for five to ten seconds. You may partially or completely lose your erection, but, then restart the stimulation and you will regain it.

Do this stop/start technique at least three times during the early stages of excitement and then continue stimulation until you ejaculate.

Don't try to control ejaculation at this point. Just concentrate on the "tickling" as you get close. The purpose of this step is to help you begin to spread control throughout the entire cycle, not just at the end.

## Step 3

The next step is a continuation of the previous step, that is three stops in the very early stages, but now, begin to add stops immediately prior to the "tickling stage".

If you look at figure 4, it may clarify what I am suggesting. Three stops very early then three stops very late. As you add the later stops, you may find that you have gone too far and you ejaculate. That is to be expected. Remember the "accidents" you had while learning bladder control.

Remember, everyone learns at a different rate. Do not get down on yourself. If you continue to practice you will get it. Continue to add to stops near the point of no return until you have reached six.

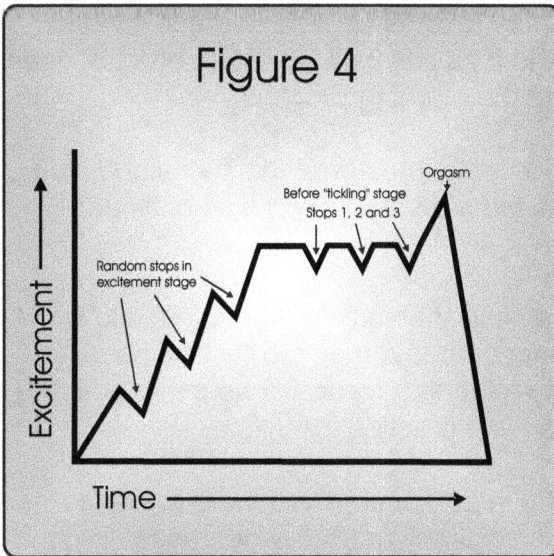

Figure 4

*Excitement* (vertical axis)

*Time* (horizontal axis)

Random stops in excitement stage

Before "tickling" stage
Stops 1, 2 and 3

Orgasm

## Step 4

This step is only necessary for some men. Up until now I have suggested that you masturbate in your usual way. For some men, this is by rubbing their pelvis against the bed or a pillow. To make this learning process most effective, it is best to masturbate in a way that mimics intercourse as closely as possible. That is, by wrapping your hand around the shaft of your penis and moving it up and down, simulating the action of the penis in the vagina. Using a lubricant can be helpful. Saliva is always available or any of the commercially marketed lubricants will do. If this technique is new for you, it may take some time to make it work. Stick with it as it is well worth the effort, it does facilitate the learning process.

Once you have mastered this technique, you can use the stop/start regime as outlined above.

You may find that initially when you follow these steps, that you go too far and have difficulty regaining control. Two things will occur as you practice.

First, the length of time you have to wait to regain control will gradually decrease. Second, the length of time you can continue stimulation between stops will increase.

As you do the exercises, remember these tips.

Keep your attention focused on the physical sensations. Remember to catch yourself when you drift into your head. Whether it is to fantasy, or to worrying about whether this process is actually working. Also, keep the chart in figure 4 in the back of your mind and try to imagine yourself following the curve.

As you continue with these exercises you will become more confident in your sense of control. Regardless of whether you have a partner or not, start with these four steps and stay with them until you have good control with self-stimulation.

I mentioned that having fantasies can distract from focusing on the physical sensations, and this is factual. However, it is often necessary to drift in and out of fantasy to maintain arousal. If you do so, I would strongly encourage you to restrict fantasies to those of thrusting with intercourse or having your partner perform oral sex on you.

Once you are confident of your control alone, it is time to bring in your partner.

## EXERCISES WITH YOUR PARTNER

As mentioned earlier, anxiety is one of the most serious impediments to learning control. It may also sabotage the gains you are making. Here is one way to eliminate as much anxiety as possible for the purpose of these exercises.

Make sure you stimulate your partner until they are satisfied (orgasm or not) BEFORE you start the exercises together. Use manual stimulation, oral stimulation or a vibrator. In that way you will not be worrying about leaving them "hanging" if you come too quickly. You will be able to concentrate more intently on your own physical sensations. Following this practice any time you have sex can help to eliminate two issues that have created problems for both men and women.

The first is the myth that in order for intercourse to be really satisfying, both partners must come at the same time. I can't estimate the number of couples I have seen over the years who come to see me because of this "problem" They've been having satisfying sex and both are having great orgasms. But, because they are not happening at exactly the same moment, they feel they are failing.

Although, the usual fairytale description of the ideal sexual encounter includes simultaneous orgasm, let me reassure you that it is rare. There are so many factors involved, for each person, that contribute to the timing of an orgasm that it almost never happens. Letting go of this myth as one of your goals will add tremendously to your enjoyment of sex.

The second myth of orgasm is even more prevalent and far more destructive. It says that if both partners do not have an orgasm with intercourse, (even if they have an orgasm with another form of stimulation), they have failed. Their experience has been "second best".

Men have told me forever, that they should be able to make a woman come with their penis. If they can't, it is because they are too small or they don't know how to use it right. What a crock!

Studies indicate that as many as seventy percent of women are unable to have an orgasm with intercourse. As I mentioned before, the equipment was designed to produce babies, not orgasm.

The clitoris is responsible for most of the stimulation that produces orgasm in women. It contains the same concentration of pleasurable nerve endings as the penis does in a man.

For most women the clitoris simply does not get enough stimulation during intercourse. The clitoris is not right next to the vagina. In some cases it is quite far away. Therefore, the penis moving in and out of the vagina does not deliver stimulation to the clitoris very well. The distance explains why some women are able to have orgasm with intercourse (when it is very close) and others can't. Regardless of how long intercourse continues. Where the distance is quite far, they will not come they will just get sore.

This also explains why some women are able to orgasm with intercourse only when they are on top. In that position they are able to get the greatest amount of stimulation delivered to the clitoris.

Once both partners accept the fact that orgasm for the woman may never occur with intercourse, they can stop feeling inadequate and get down to finding other ways to get her there. Understanding the absurdity of these two myths will reduce the pressure on you during the exercises.

In addition, as you become more comfortable with the concept, you may decide, that even after you have developed control, you will want to continue the practice. Particularly if your partner is one of the many women who do not reach orgasm with intercourse.

## Step 1

We left the exercises with you stimulating yourself, stopping a couple of times randomly early in the cycle and then stopping six times as you approached the point of no return. Now your partner begins to do exactly the same thing. Of course, you will have to tell them when and for how long to stop. As you transition to the partner exercises, expect to lose some of the control you have been developing by yourself. Work at catching yourself when you are in your head worrying about what is going on for them, and bring your attention back to your physical sensations.

## Step 2

In this step you are going to do the same thing as in step 1, only have your partner use a lubricant, which makes it more stimulating and feels more like the vaginal environment.

## Step 3

In this step, in order to further simulate the excitement of the vaginal environment, oral sex is included. But, whether or not a couple includes this step will depend on how comfortable both partners feel about oral sex. Attitudes in the last decade or two, particularly among younger men and women, have changed significantly.

What was seen as taboo and "kinky" by many, has become more  mainstream and accepted as a normal part of most couples sexual repertoire. As with the addition of lubricant in the previous step, oral stimulation more closely mimics the vaginal environment. It is warm and wet, so that the amount of stimulation to the penis is even greater. Once again, follow the same pattern; a couple of random stops in the early stage of excitement followed by stops nearer and nearer to the point of no return. Increase up to six stops before ejaculating.

## Step. 4

If your partner is female, begin with one of the previous steps, but then, have her guide your penis into her vagina. Use a lot of lubricant to ensure easy entry. She should do this while sitting astride your thighs and facing you. In that position she can easily lift herself up, guide entry, and control the speed at which she lowers herself down onto you. Be aware that for some of you, it may take a number of attempts before full entry is achieved without ejaculating. Even though you have been able to control for considerable periods with manual and/or oral stimulation in the previous exercises, this step, may be difficult for you.

Once you have achieved full entry, remain absolutely motionless,

Focus your full attention on the sensations of vaginal containment for three minutes. Once you have been able to do this on three separate occasions you are ready for the next step. If you are able to accomplish this step on the first try without difficulty, it is going to be tempting to rush ahead. I want to encourage you in the strongest terms not to! Stay with the steps, and you will not be disappointed.

## Step 5

The next step is to initiate movement. But, there are some things to remember. Let your partner do all the moving. Your job is to simply lie on your back, concentrating on the sensations in your penis, upper thighs, and lower abdomen as she begin to slowly lift herself up, then lower herself down. You tell her how quickly to move, and when to stop and start. Follow the same pattern of a few stops early in the cycle, followed by stops that get closer and closer to the point of no return. As you feel yourself approaching ejaculation, signal her to stop moving. She should not withdraw but simply stop moving. Once you are back in control, she can begin to move again. Just as with manual stimulation, you will find that, gradually the length of time you have to wait to regain control gets shorter and the length of time between stops gets longer. Continue until you are able to stop six times before going on to ejaculate.

## Step 6

This is identical to Step 5, only now, you begin to move slowly with your partner. She remains on top, so, the amount of moving you can do is limited. You then gradually increase the amount of movement with each session. As you start to move, it becomes more difficult to limit your attention to the physical sensations in your body. The temptation to drift into your head, to observe yourself and your partner, will become stronger. Once again, each time you catch yourself doing so, gently bring your focus back to the physical. In the back of your mind, keep an image of yourself on the curve.

## Step 7

Repeat the previous step, only now do so lying on your sides facing each other. This allows you a little more ability to move, yet still restricts full pelvic thrusting.
Do not get upset if you find that as you move through these steps, with each new position, your ability to control slips. With some of the transitions it may be minimal, while with others it may be significant.

## Step 8

The final position is with you on top. The majority of men have most difficulty controlling in this position. The reason is that pelvic thrusting tends to trigger the ejaculatory reflex. If you are having serious difficulty with this position, here is a suggestion that may be helpful.

When you are supporting yourself on your hands and knees, there are two ways that you can move your penis in and out. The first is by rocking your entire body back and forth. Your pelvis (with attached penis) will move back and forward along with your chest, abdomen and legs. The second way to move your penis in and out is by tilting your pelvis back and forth (thrusting), without moving the rest of your body. This is the movement that tends to trigger the ejaculatory reflex.

Limiting the amount of pelvic thrusting initially may help you make the transition in this final stage.

Well, that's it. Following these steps will work.

Be sure to give yourself some appreciation for every small success and don't get down on yourself for progressing too slowly. Keep practicing and you will get it.

# FOR THE PARTNERS

In closing, I would like to address two issues that have been raised on many occasions by the partners of clients. One is a question about the process, and the other a criticism of it. The question most often asked by partners is, of course, "How can I best help my partner with the program?" "What can I do to speed up his progress and what should I not be doing that would slow it down?"

The single most important thing you can do is to encourage him to work at it as frequently as possible. Be available to work with him when you are able, even though at times it feels like a chore, and encourage him to work on it alone when you are not available.

The second thing is to ensure that he is feeling as little pressure as possible. You do not have to pretend to be overjoyed about going through this process, but do reassure him that you are there because you want to be - for the relationship. Let him know that you realize the benefits this will bring to both of you. You may have to convince him that you can have a great experience without having an orgasm with intercourse. And you may have to convince him that an orgasm with other forms of stimulation can be totally satisfying.

Remember, you are going to have to reassure him of these things many times before he really believes you.

The criticism I hear most often is; "Where is the feeling in all this? The romance? The passion? The love?" "It all seems so mechanical. Your insistence on staying with the physical doesn't leave any room for feeling". "I don't want a partner who can last forever if the result is that he has become a machine."

I understand these concerns completely and agree that they are valid. Let me assure you that this is not going to happen. This program is a time-limited experience. It is designed to teach men to develop control in the same way they learned to control their bladders. Once they have learned, they no longer have to focus on the physical in the same way. They no longer have to think about it.

Once they are confident of control, they have the freedom to explore all dimensions of the sexual experience. Playful, sensual, emotional and spiritual.

# SUMMARY

## Solo Exercises

1. Learn to recognize the sensations that precede ejaculation.
2. Stop and start randomly during early excitement.
3. Stop and start as you near the point of no return. Work up to six stops before ejaculating.
4. Learn to ejaculate by stoking shaft of penis.
5. Include use of lubricant.

## Partner Exercises

1. Partner provides manual stimulation with stops and starts.
2. Partner adds use of lubricant.
3. Partner provides oral stimulation with stops and starts.
4. Partner guides penile insertion. No movement.
5. Partner begins slow movement with stops and starts.
6. Male begins to move slowly.
7. Continue to start and stop in lateral position.
8. Male assumes superior position and fully controls stops and starts.

www.ingramcontent.com/pod-product-compliance
Lightning Source LLC
LaVergne TN
LVHW021547080426
835509LV00019B/2890